Helping Children Form Healthy Attachments

For our children: Aster, Saul, Galina,
Maarten, Michaela, Mariza

Translated by Barbara Mees

First published in Dutch as *Gezond hechten* by Uitgeverij
Christofoor in 2015
First published in English by Floris Books in 2017
© 2015 Uitgeverij Christofoor, Zeist
English version © 2017 Floris Books

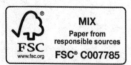

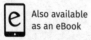

Also available
as an eBook

British Library CIP data available
ISBN 978-178250-372-9
Printed in Great Britain
by Bell & Bain, Ltd

Helping Children Form Healthy Attachments

Building the Foundation for
Strong Lifelong Relationships

Loïs Eijgenraam

Floris
Books

Contents

Part 1.
What is Healthy
Attachment?

1. Healthy Attachments for Harmonious Living

We are all meant to shine, as children do. We were born to make manifest the glory of God that is within us. It is not just in some of us; it is in everyone.

Marianne Williamson, *A Return to Love*

The term 'healthy attachment' refers to the bonds children form within themselves and with the world around them. Being 'healthily attached' involves feeling safe, at ease, being able to trust others, having self-confidence and the confidence to explore. Bonding with ourselves is the foundation for building relationships with parents, carers, friends, even with plants and animals – in short, with the entire world.

This book is about the process of becoming healthily attached, giving insight into how healthy attachment develops, the conditions required for successful bonding and how parents, carers and educators can help. A number of influences in my life inspired me to explore the process of healthy attachment in young children.

When I became a mother in 1989, I started to look into the process of bonding as part of my broader aim of learning how to live 'in harmony' with my children. This goal then extended to living harmoniously with all the other people in my life, as well as with the earth, animals – even the sun, moon and stars, which form part of this harmony, as does our culture with its festivals and traditions. I started to make conscious choices about how our family could live more harmoniously within our world: this meant choices about the furnishings in our home, about toys that the children received or didn't receive, about nutrition and mealtimes, about how to spend free time and holidays, about children's clothes, about illness, medications and cosmetics; it seemed that everything was intertwined.

During my years as a kindergarten teacher in a Steiner-Waldorf school and a tutor at the Academy for Parents, I found that many parents had concerns and questions about raising their children. For example, they might ask how to provide security and structure in children's upbringing; how to deal with parental differences of opinion; how to set boundaries for children and how many boundaries are required; how to be consistent in parenting, which is not always easy. Another common theme was balancing work with raising young children: 'If my child goes to day care does that make me a lesser parent than someone who is at home full-time?' Feelings of guilt such as this often go hand in hand with parents' high expectations or ideals. But such thoughts can be paralysing and may prevent us from finding a helpful solution to the problem. Being open and honest about such feelings within ourselves and with others can help us to explore and address such issues.

I also had the privilege to meet families whose nurturing approach to the attachment process showed a great deal of love and warmth. These parents – often a mother and father, but also single parents or same-sex parents – understood and utilised the building blocks needed to create a life-long foundation for their children.

They were educators who took responsibility for their own biography, meaning that they were aware of patterns brought with them from their own childhood, and they were conscious that these patterns could sometimes get in the way. For example, during one of my courses a father explained that his own father was very quick-tempered. As a child, if he did something that annoyed him, he would yell or slam his fist on the table. His father could never speak calmly about what made him angry. During the course this father said that he, as a parent, also found it difficult to suppress anger. At the same time, he found himself being too lenient towards his child, thus doing the opposite of his father's example. By working with a biographer and psychologist, he was able to deal with these childhood issues and break the pattern. He took responsibility for his own biography and consciously tried to raise his own children differently. Struggling to find parenting answers in our own upbringings was a common theme: our lifestyle has changed so much that those examples often don't seem relevant to today's society (see Chapter 2, p.17).

Another observation I made during courses with Steiner-Waldorf parents was how well many of them tune in to the needs of their children. They are always there for their children, even amid the flurry of their hectic lives. They are fully present during everything they do with their children at a given moment; taking a walk as a family means actually walking and talking, not also checking email or social media on their phone along the way. They are aware of what is age-appropriate for their children and can support and empathise on a suitable level. If we look closely at children and what makes and keeps them healthy, we will find the answers to our parenting questions in children themselves. Through careful observation we can develop a sensitive internal instrument tuned to the needs of a specific child.

These parents set boundaries that are fitting to the age and capabilities of their children. And they explain rules clearly: when we eat, there are no books or toys on the table; we always try a small bite of something that we don't know or don't like.

Through my work in Steiner-Waldorf schools, I learned about the senses and how they work together to enable health, growth, movement, and our human need to play and explore. When we speak about the senses, we often mean the five senses: of sight, touch, hearing, smell and taste. But Rudolf Steiner, the Austrian philosopher who developed the theory behind Steiner-Waldorf education, described twelve senses: touch, life, movement, balance, smell, taste, sight, warmth, hearing, speech, thought and self (or other). Broadening our understanding of the senses in this way gives us much deeper insight into human experiences. In this book we will look closely at the senses of touch, life, movement and balance.

I have also met families who were affected by domestic violence, addiction, neglect, or emotional or sexual abuse. A few times children in my class were labelled COPMI (Child of Parent with a Mental Illness) by social workers. In these less stable family situations, social workers and all those involved had to continually assess how to best care for these children, and whether they should continue living at home or whether they would have a healthier childhood if placed in a temporary foster home. According to my own experience, these children appeal to their surroundings to provide the building blocks needed for attachment (described fully in Part 2). It is vitally important that these children have people around them who are willing to show them love, to be there for them, and to create a home that is stable and healthy.

I am an advocate of education through hope, no matter how hard the circumstances are. Everyone should encounter love through *one* human being who continues to believe in them and in their power to fulfil their destiny in this world. This may be a neighbour, a teacher, the school janitor or someone they just happen to meet. One person can make all the difference in another person's biography.

If you treat an individual as he is, he will remain how he is. But if you treat him as if he were what he ought to be and could be, he will become what he ought to be and could be.

Goethe

I wrote this book to help parents, caregivers and educators develop healthy relationships with children, enabling those in their care to build strong foundations for life ahead. Tuning in closely to the needs of our children and supporting them effectively will, in turn, help us to live harmoniously with other family members and with those around us.

To quote a key statement from the charity Unicef: 'A world fit for children, is a world fit for everyone.' (Unicef, Millennium Development Goals)

The following verse embodies the vision we will explore in this book in relation to healthy attachment.

*Childhood is a time for learning about
the essentials –
about the heavenly world and the earthly,
about goodness, beauty and truth.*

*Childhood is a time to be loved and to love –
to express fear and to learn trust –
to be allowed to be serious and calm
and to celebrate with laughter and joy.*

*Children have a right to dream,
and they need time to grow at their own pace.
They have the right to make mistakes
and the right to be forgiven.*

*Children need to help to develop self-mastery,
to transform themselves and bring forth
their highest capacities.
Children have a right to be spared violence and
hunger,
to have a home and protection.
They need help to grow up healthily,
with good habits and sound nutrition.*

*Children need people to respect,
adults whose example and loving authority
they follow.
They need a range of experience –
tenderness and kindness,
boldness and courage, and even mischief
and misbehaviour.*

*Children need time for receiving and giving,
for belonging and participating.
They need to be part of a community,
and they need to be individuals.
They need privacy and sociability.
They need time to rest and time to play,
time to do nothing and time to work.*

*They need moments for devotion and room
for curiosity.
They need protective boundaries and freedom
for creativity.
They need to be introduced to a life
of principles
and given the freedom to discover their own.
They need a relationship to the earth –
to animals and to nature,
and they need to unfold as human beings
within the community.*

*The spirit of childhood is to be protected
and nurtured.
It is an essential part of every human being
and needs to be kept alive.*

International Joint Alliance Working Group,
New York, 1999

2. A Brief History of Parenting in the Twentieth Century

Our task is to thankfully connect to our past and to trust in the future.

Rudolf Meyer

In many parts of Western Europe people's lives have changed enormously over the past hundred years. Let's think back to the 1920s, when many people lived in the villages or towns where their parents and grandparents had been born and raised. The population was divided into religious groups, such as Roman Catholics and Protestants, and lifestyle was stipulated for the most part by the church. Men tended to work outside the home, whereas wives and mothers tended to stay at home doing housework, caring for children and sometimes working for the family business. The discovery of penicillin in 1928 meant that the death rate decreased, in both adults and children.

During the 1920s it was commonly accepted that children needed rest, good hygiene and a clear routine. People believed that if children were cuddled, they would not become independent or respect their elders. Parents shook their children by the hand and routine was considered of paramount importance: church on Sunday, laundry on Monday, ironing on Tuesday, storytelling on Wednesday, and so on. Children were disciplined by physical punishment, and this was even preached in church: 'He that spareth his rod hateth his son.' (Book of Proverbs 13:24)

The Second World War can be seen as a turning point for many long-standing traditions and habits. From 1945 onwards people in Europe and around the world were so busy rebuilding their countries that they had little time to reflect on the grief and trauma that surrounded them. Raising children effectively meant teaching them to be strong, not to cry and not to ask for help from others, which was generally seen as a weakness.

In 1946 Dr Benjamin Spock published his book *Baby and Child Care*, which caused a revolution in childcare. He advocated cuddling and encouraged parents to respond individually to the unique needs of their children, since all children develop and respond in their own special way.

In the 1970s parents were advised to pick their children up and comfort them when they cried, because babies need love, familiarity and emotional space. But this perspective presented new mothers with a challenge, being in stark contradiction to advice from their own mothers, who had learned that crying helped develop the lungs. In the following years advice changed again:

suggesting that we let children cry for a little while before comforting them.

Today, in our increasingly digital world, there's a huge range of differing perspectives on parenting. Advice is constantly evolving and being presented to parents, who then have to decide for themselves which stance best suits their lifestyle and ideals. Advice on setting boundaries, saying no and knowing what is 'right for the child', for example, is not as clear as it once was. Some movements believe we should discuss everything with our children; others say parents should give firm guidance until a certain age; others that children should be allowed freedom to develop themselves from as early an age as possible.

And so ideas go back and forth, but what seems consistent over the years is that the vast majority of parents, and society as a whole, have the best interests of children in mind; in fact we are all looking for ways to bond successfully, for points of attachment.

In reality, all children develop in their own unique way, at their own unique pace. Many children start taking their first steps around their first birthday, some start walking at nine months and others don't start until they are twenty months. Parents who have a sensitive relationship with their child know intuitively if there's reason to be concerned. Advice about child development is necessary and interesting, but no one child follows generalised developmental patterns to the letter. Parents should observe their children as they walk their own unique path of development.

Social change

The older generations today will still remember times when key social figures, such as priests and headmasters, had a huge influence on the way people lived their lives. Today we have much more freedom to determine our own lifestyle choices. Through the wealth of media that surrounds us, all manner of information is available at the touch of a button or swipe of a screen – something unavailable to our parents' generation.

Scientists are constantly analysing how the human body functions, which provides new insight into child-development and in turn to our parenting choices. For example, the discovery of mirror neurons has shown us that humans imitate, copy and sympathise visibly and invisibly, which is an important discovery in relation to child development: children copy their caregivers in almost everything they do. Young children look for gestures, words and movements, and copy them. For example, in one family one child may copy the mother's facial expressions while another copies the way the father walks. As children grow older (7–21 years of age) they look for aspirational figures to model or take inspiration from. For example, a seven-year-old wants to learn to read and write 'just like Mrs Jones'; a fourteen-year-old wants to hear her teacher's answers to 'life's questions' – the teacher has become an aspirational figure who guides the youngster on her path in life through telling stories and offering personal examples with which the child can identify.

In recent decades we've also seen significant change in terms of our development as human beings – one physical example being our sense of self-awareness. Until the 1980s, we generalised that children become self-aware and first start to use the word 'I' around their third year. Nowadays, children often say and mean 'I' before they are two-and-a-half years old. The process of individualisation is happening earlier. Children who say 'I' at a young age appeal for secure attachments with their caregivers even more so than those who become self-aware slightly later, since the body, which will become the home of the 'I', is less developed than that of a three-year-old. The attachment process has therefore become even more vulnerable in recent years.

Many of the building blocks on which adults built their lives in the early twentieth century, such as the church, the perceived roles of men and women, sources of energy, transport and communication have changed dramatically. I believe that the building blocks with which we create the foundations of our lives in today's society can be found in the following principles: routine in our daily lives, living with the rhythm of the seasons, respect, finding a balance between rest and activity, security, diligence, carving out enough 'me time', creativity, responsibility and autonomy.

3. The Beginnings of Attachment Theory

Even if I knew that tomorrow the world would go to pieces, I would still plant my apple tree.

Martin Luther

I didn't encounter the subject of healthy attachment as a student, but it has increasingly been brought to our attention in recent years. The English psychiatrist John Bowlby (1907–1990), in particular, carried out significant research into the bonding process between parents and their carers. He was asked by the World Health Organisation (WHO) to carry out research on many children who had been taken into orphanages during the Second World War. It had come to the attention of the WHO that the behaviour of many of these children differed from that of children who were raised at home by their parents or others they were close to.

Babies who were placed in orphanages during their first year commonly displayed either fierce opposition – in the form of anger, aggression to others and themselves, and inconsolable crying – or serious apathy towards their new carers, closing themselves off from their surroundings and not seeking contact. They didn't play with other children, showed no appetite and stared apathetically into the world. The development of these children seemed to have been disrupted.

Bowlby first thought this behaviour was due to a lack of motherly love, which he believed was as important to child development as vitamins and proteins. He later revised his theory, to hypothesise that children were becoming detached due to the lack of a key figure with whom to bond, rather than due to the absence of a mother in particular. Orphanages were chronically short of staff and those they had were overworked and still trying to process the tragedy of war themselves, with all its emotional consequences. Orphanage staff didn't have the time or inner peace to develop trusting relationships with individual children.

Between 1945 and 1950 Bowlby expanded his research and the concept of bonding and 'attachment theory' became part of developmental psychology. Bowlby's research gave insight into two key aspects of the process of healthy bonding:

1. Personal orientation, manifested in feelings of self-confidence and autonomy.
2. Orientation towards others, manifested in feelings of basic safety and trusting others.

Bowlby discovered four phases in the bonding process:

- Phase 1: basic safety (connected to the sense of touch in this book) – if children don't feel safe, they develop fear.
- Phase 2: trust (connected to the sense of life in this book) – if children don't have faith in those around them, they'll be unable to trust others.
- Phase 3: self-confidence (connected to the sense of movement in this book) – without self-confidence, children feel insecure.
- Phase 4: freedom (connected to the sense of balance in this book) – without freedom, children feel lonely.

Furthermore, Bowlby categorised a number of important aspects of the process of bonding by age:

- 0–3 months: the first phase in which babies must adapt to their surroundings and find a new balance.
- 3–6 months: during this period the first psychological bonding occurs. We now speak of a symbiotic relationship between child and parent, parent and child.
- 6–36 months: the phase of individualisation and separation. Children typically look for proximity with a carer, before distancing themselves again. At the end of the second year we see the rebellious 'terrible twos'. During the third year the first psychological birth of the 'I' occurs.

- 36 months onwards: the process of attachment and detachment continues throughout life.

Guilt

It was only after much critique and extended research that Bowlby adjusted his first conclusion – that orphans were experiencing psychological issues and developmental delay due to a lack of motherly love – to an absence of someone with whom to bond.

Around the same time, research into autism was underway. One of the first proposed explanations for autism was that autistic children must have what were termed 'refrigerator mothers', who were emotionally distant, leading their children in turn to become emotionally detached and difficult. It soon became apparent that this conclusion was also incorrect.

Unreliable research such as this can have the negative effect of making parents, especially mothers, feel under pressure and even guilty about the way they raise their children. Even in our time, certain subjects and uncertainties – such as attachment and whether or not to vaccinate children – often ignite feelings of guilt in parents. There are no clear-cut answers. As parents we must face the challenge, gather all the necessary information, then form our own ideas and opinions.

4. It Takes a Whole Village to Raise a Child

Man's goodness is a flame that can be hidden but never extinguished.

Nelson Mandela, *Long Walk to Freedom*

When children are raised by two parents, they are likely to build close bonds with them both. Children may also develop a close bond with just one parent or with another adult with whom they have a long-standing relationship.

However, children don't always form healthy bonds with both parents. Sometimes attachment develops with one parent but not the other, especially if the weaker relationship hasn't been built on strong foundations using the building blocks we will go on to discuss in Part 2 of safety, trust, self-confidence, independence and creativity. It could be that one parent has a more sensitive approach to the child than the other. In times of stress or fear children will reach out to the carer with whom they are most securely attached.

I have found that parents who struggle to bond with their children are often struggling to come to terms with attachment problems during their own childhood. If that's the case, it's important to recognise these issues and work through them. In this instance it can be challenging to support each other as partners, but the primary goal must be to raise children in as healthy a manner as possible (see Chapter 1, p.11 for more on taking responsibility for our own biographies).

But it's not only the primary caregivers who are involved in the process of raising healthy, happy children. The title of this chapter comes from an African saying that has proved key in answering many of the questions put to me by parents and caregivers. It asserts that several people are needed to raise a healthy child – a whole village – and the choice of this word is important. Unlike a city, in a traditional African village a group of people live and work together closely; they know each other well. Life in the village is well balanced, with people dividing tasks and responsibilities effectively between them. All aspects of the village – the houses, streets and facilities – are in proportion and regularly adapted to suit the requirements of the people living there.

Similarly, parents and caregivers look for and rely upon a group of people who interact closely to function as a 'village' for their children. This may include carers at playgroup or kindergarten; it may include other parents who take turns caring for children while other parents are at work; it will almost certainly include close friends and family.

The younger the child, the smaller the village. For young babies 'the village' is the home, garden and neighbourhood in which walks are taken; for toddlers, it may be extended to playschool or day care; then to kindergarten or primary school, which marks the first significant step into the 'big, wide world' – a world in which children will begin to live their own lives, no longer so tightly tied to home. Children sometimes spend more waking hours at school than they do at home.

The village is not passive. It grows alongside children and their parents. The most important aspect of a child's village is that the inhabitants all know one another, that they share a similar approach to raising children and that they can communicate effectively.

But of course children perceive all members of their village differently, and some may play a significant role in children's lives without developing a close attachment.

The difference between an attachment figure and a trusted figure

The principal attachment figures in children's lives are usually their primary caregivers, whether they be a mother, father, step-parent or other carer. Both children and adults become securely attached to people with whom we develop long-standing emotional bonds.

A trusted figure may play an important role in a child's life, and may influence the rest of that child's life. It may be someone who enters their life only once, but has a big impact; or, it could be someone who visits regularly, such as a grandmother who comes to visit her grandson once a month: the child enjoys sharing experiences with her, trusts her and feels supported by her. Children often share a trusting relationship with their teacher, particularly if they have the same class teacher for a number of years. Depending on the number of days a toddler attends childcare and the changes in personnel, a key care worker may fulfil this role.

Support staff at school may become key trusted figures. For example, a ten-year-old girl was referred for extra support at school because of low academic achievement and social withdrawal following problems at home. A psychologist spent one day with the child – an expert who understood her situation, knew which questions to ask, and was able to pinpoint the problem. The girl opened up to the psychologist about life at home and bullying in the classroom. She felt so comfortable with the psychologist that this trusted figure with whom she had only spent one day was able to make a difference for her entire school life.

Most people have trusted figures we can call on at any time; times of stress tend to reveal who these people are. Trusted figures make a significant impact and lasting memories throughout life. For example, we may remember a friend who took one of our toys (3 years old), going to the doctor or the dentist (4 years and older), our first romantic relationship (16 years old).

Working together

Without making a judgement, nor making parents or educators feel guilty, I believe children ask those in their 'village' for a loving and intensive collaboration. In reality, toddlers and preschool children are raised by more than just one or two people, and the attachment process concerns them all, not only the parents.

It seems that today's children ask us (completely unconsciously): Could you please work together as much as possible? Could you show me through your words and actions how to create healthy bonds, so that I can imitate you? If I can imitate you, I can grow into a loving, independent person who can take and give responsibility; a person who can care and be cared for, who can support and sympathise, who is strong and clear, who can trust completely and be completely trusted in this world.

Part 2.
Building Blocks
in the Attachment
Process

5. The Attachment Pyramid

If you want to get somewhere quickly, go alone. If you want to go far, go together.

Mathias Wais

The process of healthy attachment involves developing relationships with ourselves, within our own bodies and with our surroundings. It does not happen spontaneously, but has specific requirements. In the following chapters I will discuss in detail how the attachment process develops, based on the work of psychotherapist Truus Bakker-van Zeil, who developed a useful diagram called the 'attachment pyramid' (see p.39), which is made up of five key 'building blocks' of child development. I was also inspired by Marijke Bijloo, special needs educationist (1955–2010), who extended the pyramid by connecting it to the senses of touch, life, movement and balance, as identified by Rudolf Steiner (see Chapter 1, p.12). I will also use Marijke Bijlloo's age classifications in my discussion.

The building blocks of attachment

I have already introduced the concept of the 'building

blocks' of healthy attachment (see Chapters 3 and 4). In the following chapters we will look at each building block in more detail, and explore how children's homes (their body) and villages (their family, neighbourhood, childcare, school, etc.) are involved in the attachment process.

In examining each building block, I will pay particular attention to the senses of touch, life, movement and balance, which allow children to experience the following:

The *sense of touch* lets children physically feel that they have their own body, in which they feel safe and protected: it is my home.

The *sense of life* allows children to experience how things stand with regards to their body: am I in harmony, do I feel comfortable in my home? I *am* my body. I dare to entrust myself with what I experience in and on my body.

The *sense of movement* enables children to live in their own body through movement and being emotionally 'moved'. Children experience a sense of freedom in and through their body, which gives them self-confidence: I am not restricted, I can move freely.

The *sense of balance* lets children experience that their self or 'I' enters the outside world: I am unique, there's only one of me in the world. When children can stand up straight and stay balanced, both in body and in spirit, they experience a sense of independence: I can stand on my own.

The development of creativity tops the development

of the senses, and the attachment pyramid, like a crown. Children can now interact with others and play, work, live and learn together.

Graphs and diagrams have pros and cons: one pro is that information is easy to access; one con is that it can lead to rigidity and pigeonholing. In the diagram above, children and parents/carers are positioned side by side – child in a box, carer in a box: not a true representation of reality, in which many arrows and threads are woven together in the complex relationships between parents and their children.

The senses discussed alongside each building block do not work in isolation; they move through one another. Each building block includes conditions that should be completely or partially met, and each time we will discuss what happens if these conditions are not attained. For example, in Building Block 1: Basic Security, if a parent consistently neglects a baby in their first year, the child will develop fear. This book focuses on the process of healthy attachment, and does not look in detail at the outcomes of insecure attachment in extreme situations such as neglect. However, everyone reading this book will recognise feelings of fear, distrust, insecurity and loneliness, to some degree. This is because no one is or has grown up being one hundred per cent safe and securely attached. The majority of parents and caregivers do their utmost but everyone makes mistakes.

I believe that everyone is born with a plan, a purpose, and that this plan includes material with which we must work and remould as we progress through life. The attachment process, therefore, does not only concern children but also adults. It is about human beings of all ages, young and old, from all over the world, from each social group, gender and race working together. Whenever I feel afraid, I look closely at the situation I have found myself in and ask: What does this person mean? Why is she angry with me? I explore the situation – I become an explorer. And then I look for support.

The attachment pyramid summarises child development in a number of phases, which we will discuss further over the following chapters. It indicates:

1. Primary age range in which children develop this building block.
2. Which sense in particular is used during each phase of development.
3. What children should do in order to develop each building block.
4. What caregivers should provide to enable children to develop healthily.
5. How children will react if their needs are not met.
6. Parental behaviour that will lead to such a negative reaction.

Child ↑	Parent/carer ↑
Creativity	**Having confidence**
1. 4–5 years old	
2. All senses	
3. Solving problems independently and with others, showing empathy, role play	4. Having confidence in our children, letting go in full faith
5. Incapable	6. Being fearful/anxious
Independence	**Strong and clear**
1. 3–4 years old	
2. Sense of balance	
3. Aware that they can do things by themselves, saying 'I', being able to form an inner image of another person, concentration, giving and taking	4. Giving children more personal space, using the word 'I', setting boundaries without rejecting, giving guidance
5. Loneliness	6. Being vague
Self-confidence	**Support and compassion**
1. 1–3 years old	
2. Sense of movement	
3. Exploring the world, dealing with separation anxiety, sharing joy and sadness, controlling emotions	4. Providing support and stimulation, compassion and understanding; letting children explore, naming things
5. Insecurity	6. Indifference or over supervision
Trust	**Giving**
1. 0–1 year old	
2. Sense of life (well-being and harmony)	
3. Surrender, daring to open up to someone or something	4. Being caring and sympathetic; watching, following, and mirroring children; talking and babbling with them, naming things
5. Distrust	6. Being selfish/taking
Basic security	**Taking responsibility, caring**
1. Pregnancy to 1 year old	
2. Sense of touch	
3. A phase of unconscious feeling, being allowed to exist, having a place, feeling comfortable and at home	4. Good living conditions, taking the lead, reacting to children's needs and signals, physical contact, love
5. Fear	6. Neglect
Child ↑	**Parent/carer ↑**

6. One: Building Basic Security

The biggest evil is when man forgets his inner kingship.

Martin Buber

Child	Parent/carer
Basic security	Taking responsibility, caring
1. Pregnancy to 1 year old	
2. Sense of touch	
3. A phase of unconscious feeling, being allowed to exist, having a place, feeling comfortable and at home	4. Good living conditions, taking the lead, reacting to children's needs and signals, physical contact, love
5. Fear	6. Neglect

The requirements needed to construct the first building block of basic security – feeling welcome, proud of one's self, protected, warm, accepted and loved – are all experienced by babies during their first nine months of life. The way in which we look after our children – how we hold them, how we care for their skin, where they sleep, how we feed them – all contribute to ensuring they feel truly welcome.

However, many factors influence our unborn children even before we meet them. These include the family situation at the time of conception, how the parents react to the pregnancy, and particularly how the mother feels throughout. The process of healthy attachment begins during pregnancy and perhaps even earlier: some parents say they can sense that a child is coming even before conception; that even before conception they lived with devotion towards their unborn child. Mother and child are deeply connected throughout the pregnancy, and ideally, she will adapt her life to best suit the requirements of her unborn child.

The relationship between the parents is also important. Does the father support the mother? Do they welcome the coming child? If the mother doesn't have a partner, are there other people to support her? The parents must work together fervently during pregnancy as this is when the first threads of attachment are woven.

In the womb, babies are surrounded by amniotic fluid and are weightless; they are intensely connected with their mother. During the birthing process, babies are rhythmically pushed through the birth canal and they are touched everywhere for the first time. Their tiny skull is powerfully 'massaged', awakening the vital functions that start developing after birth.

Following this, the umbilical cord is immediately cut from the placenta. As a reaction to this sudden feeling of breathlessness, babies begin to breathe. If we consider this from the perspective of attachment – successful arrival in the body that will become home – wouldn't it be better if the placenta were allowed to stop slowly? The last remaining blood, oxygen and nutrients would then be able to enter the body, and babies would start to breathe when ready. We have learned from experience that babies who start life in this way, and not through a feeling of breathlessness, are more in tune to their surroundings after birth.

This said, I'm aware that such a gradual introduction to this world is not possible for every parent and baby. For example, sometimes babies must be born by caesarean section. But even in that situation we can be wise, meaning: as parents we can search for a solution to a problem we didn't ask for; we can try to accept and, where possible, address and remould the situation. We might tightly swaddle a baby born by caesarean section immediately after birth, substituting some of the experience of passing through the birth canal. We might sing to this baby a lot, allowing them to experience the process of breathing in another way. Singing supports and harmonises the breathing process and, according to research, has a calming effect on children. In the case of caesarean section or any other intervention during the birthing process, parents still have the opportunity to tenderly tune in to their own child from the very beginning.

Developing the sense of touch

The sense of touch lets children experience that they have their own body. I have my body in which I experience basic safety and protection. It is my home. Touching another human being can be a deep and intense experience, sometimes giving us goose bumps or making us blush. An example of how intense the sense of touch can be is the story of Kyrie and Brielle Jackson.

They were born twelve weeks prematurely and were put in two separate incubators. Little Brielle was not well: she was struggling to breathe and her heartbeat was very weak. A nurse discussed the possibility of putting the two children in one incubator, the parents agreed and the two girls were put together. Little Kyrie immediately put her arm around Brielle and from that moment on, Brielle got stronger: her heartbeat stabilised and her water balance was restored. The girls grew quickly and when they went home, their parents placed them in the same crib. They continued to sleep close together through kindergarten. This is how intense and life saving the sense of touch can be.

The sense of touch allows us to experience the boundaries between our surroundings and ourselves: I am here and the world begins there. As the skin is the organ that feels, the sense of touch is spread over a human's entire body. Not only the skin on the outside but also the tongue and cheeks while eating or sucking.

During birth, a baby's entire body is touched by the birth canal, awakening the sense of touch. Carrying and cuddling our children further awakens their sense of touch; we hold our children not only physically but also emotionally. Children touch objects, such as toys or the side of a cot, or these objects touch them, and are physically experienced as being outside children's bodies, not part of themselves. Relatively soon, consciously knowing where the one ends and the other begins will become an important step in the development of self-awareness, the 'I'.

By being mindful of how children experience touch with regard to nature, toys, clothing, physical contact with others, and by consciously caring for what 'touches' our children's inner being, they can reach the deepest essence of this sense, which will enable them to actually meet another human being. This is not only true for children but for everyone: 'A world fit for children is a world fit for everyone!' (see p.14)

There are a number of ways in which we can encourage babies to develop their sense of touch, thereby giving them the necessary experience and parameters to feel secure in their bodies.

Rhythm

Even during pregnancy we can create predictability and routine. Before birth, babies float in the daily rhythm of their mother. Fathers can join in by resting with their partner and sharing moments of relaxation. Research has shown that the heart rates of both mother and the unborn child decrease when relaxing. Expectant mothers who rest during the day often have babies that can get used to the circadian rhythm more easily than mothers who have busy schedules or limited time to relax. Resting doesn't have to mean taking a nap, but can include meditation, taking a moment to watch the clouds pass in the sky or appreciate wild flowers in a field, or just plain staring into space.

Following birth, rest and peaceful surrounding are important to ensure young children are not overwhelmed by too many experiences at once. Predictability helps babies to develop their sense of touch and strengthens their feeling of security – familiarity of the physical objects and materials that touch their young skin, as well familiarity of our facial expressions, body language and general reactions.

You will have noticed that one thing young children cannot tolerate is haste. Trying to do anything with young children in a hurry is pointless, as their understanding of time has not yet fully developed; they live right now, in the moment. Young children teach us that routine, repetition, predictability, humour, and alternation between action and relaxation are essential ingredients in the process of healthy attachment.

When children grow older, daily activities, habits and routines develop. A preschooler knows that we always eat meals at the dining table. A kindergartner knows that we only read one picture book at bedtime. An adolescent knows that she should write her homework down in a diary. None of these habits need to be explained again every time. Habits, rhythms and routine give children, parents and teachers a foundation. These structures are not only good for children, but also for their caregivers. Everyone knows where they stand and everyone feels safe within the predictability of these habits.

Like captains of the ship, caregivers must lead this process of bringing rhythm, habit and routine into children's lives; in doing so we are helping children incarnate into their own bodies.

Rocking and the sense of balance

Many parents instinctively rock newborn babies. Whether in the arms of a parent or older sibling, rocking allows babies to experience not only the sense of touch but also the sense of balance. By sense of balance I don't mean solely the physical balance required for sitting, crawling or standing, but also emotional balance within ourselves. Children who cry and are rocked in their parents' arms re-establish this sense of balance each time they are rocked. With the support given by the parents' comfort and proximity, young children are able to develop their emotional balance, which in turn contributes to a key building block of 'being balanced' and knowing how to regain balance. A 'balanced person' is someone who doesn't become emotionally unsettled easily. Many young parents have said to me that, once their child has been comforted and is peaceful again, they themselves feel better and regain their inner balance. This is true for parents with children of all ages; nurturing the senses never stops. The emphasis on nurturing the sense of touch lies primarily in the first year of life, but toddlers, kindergartners, adolescents and the elderly in particular also need this care.

Skin-to-skin contact, vernix and skincare

Babies experience the sense of touch during and immediately following birth. Doctors and midwives often guide babies out of the birth canal before placing them on the mother's chest. This first moment of direct skin-to-skin contact between mother and child is crucial, but it's not always possible straightaway, for example, if the baby is delivered by caesarean section or needs to be examined urgently by a doctor. But parents must not feel guilty in such cases. If the mother can't hold the child immediately, a partner or family member can welcome the child with direct skin-to-skin contact and gentle stroking, or this important moment can follow after the necessary medical procedures.

Many children are born with vernix on their skin. During pregnancy, vernix nourishes the skin and prevents it from drying out. Vernix is often washed off newborn babies straight after birth, but this is a shame as it also has a function after birth: protecting against cold, infection and dehydration. It would be better for babies to leave vernix until it is fully absorbed by the skin.

Children's skin needs daily care until approximately their fourth year, while the epidermis develops. Natural oils are easily absorbed by young children's skin and allow the skin to 'breathe'. Taking time to consciously massage babies and young children also cares for their sense of touch.

In winter and summer it's also important to protect the skin from excessive cold or warmth.

Swaddling

Swaddling can be very calming for newborns and sometimes even for older babies. Swaddling lets them experience boundaries: I am here and the world begins there. In doing so it helps children feel safe and secure and has a calming effect: children cry less and sleep better. As do the parents!

Although swaddling is an ancient tradition, it has not always been officially recommended, but it continues to be standard practice for many nurses, midwives and parents. It looks easy, which it is when you get the hang of it, but at the same time it's a fine art, and should neither be too loose nor too tight. You will find further information on swaddling online, or in some of the books listed in the Bibliography.

Setting Boundaries: 'Invisible swaddling cloths'

By experiencing the boundaries provided by swaddling, children feel safe and protected. Similarly the boundaries children experience in their upbringing also act as 'invisible swaddling cloths' for their social and emotional development. The caregiver understands the developmental needs and aptitudes of their children at various ages and applies appropriate boundaries or 'swaddling cloths' throughout life. For example, a two-year-old is given very limited choice and not asked to choose from five different kinds of sandwich or types of yoghurt. A kindergartner knows that only two after-school play-dates are allowed each week. An adolescent is given a set amount of time per day to spend on the computer or on social media.

Too many or too few boundaries

During the first seven years, especially until the first time the child says 'I', children have a symbiotic relationship with their parents. As the years pass, they develop an inner world in which they start to experience themselves. They need boundaries, safety and structure in order to develop their own identity within their inner self.

Adolescents and adults who experience an emotional breakdown sometimes mention that they have difficulty sensing their own boundaries or those of others. This is often because they were given too few or too many boundaries as children. They are unable to deal with or accept personal boundaries or those set by others, and struggle to accept resistance or setbacks. In other words, children need a healthy dose of Vitamin F – frustration (a kindergartner learning how to tie his shoes, an adolescent saving up for a new laptop and learning to set priorities to reach that goal); and Vitamin B – boredom (a kindergartner being content to play by himself, an adolescent being able to fill free time without always being on social media).

Children who are raised with boundaries that are 'too strict' (who are swaddled too tightly) can develop the need to step out of line, with all the consequences this may bring. In Dutch there is a saying that children are 'swaddled too hot', meaning someone is quick-tempered. This comes from times when swaddling cloths used to hang by the stove to warm. If they were hung too close to the stove, they would get too hot for the child. We can translate this saying for our own time and purpose in this book: when tending to the sense of touch and setting boundaries for our children, we must examine each instance carefully and sensitively; not too warm and not too cold, not too loose and not too tight.

Clothing

Clothing is always in contact with children's skin and so is important in developing children's sense of touch. Clothing made from natural materials (silk, wool, cotton) feel different from synthetic materials. Natural materials are breathable and allow children to learn to regulate their own perspiration. A silk or woollen beanie protects a child from losing too much heat via the head and gives extra protection from the outside world.

Children are able to understand the origins of clothes and toys made from natural materials more easily. For example, the wool of a sheep gives us warmth through the woollen clothing that we wear; therefore we all know that wool gives warmth. When children see sheep with thick fleeces in fields, the images of the warm sweater and woollen fleece and the connection between them is easy to process; it's a genuine image. Fleece sweaters, made from materials that originate from petroleum, can also be wonderfully warm and practical – but a child has no connection with petroleum and no facility to imagine the process by which it can create warmth.

Consequently, the sense of touch thrives and develops best through touching as many natural products as possible.

Inner protection: hoodies and baseball caps

Above we considered the holistic effect of swaddling cloths, both visible and invisible, and their sheathing, protective effect for babies and children. Every age group seems to have its own type of 'swaddling'. Babies feel protected when swaddled; toddlers, kindergartners and primary-school children enjoy dressing up and playing with clothes to explore their identity; children in later primary and secondary school often wear hooded sweaters and many of them love pulling the hoods over their ears. It's as if they are looking for protection from the outside world and unconsciously saying, 'Leave me in my own cocoon so I can work on my own identity.' Later on as adolescents, they may wear baseball caps, hide their hands in their sleeves and be 'not at home'. Wearing caps or hoods is not usually allowed at school because everyone is part of the larger group – no one is singled out and everyone must be seen. But parents and educators should ask themselves why children feel the need for this extra layer of protection.

How parents can help

Take a minute to ask yourself: How do I deal with

experiences involving the sense of touch? In which situations do I sense or build boundaries? When do I feel safe and unsafe? Have I set too many boundaries for my children, which may limit their space to develop? In other words: In which situations do I 'overprotect'?

Parents can develop the sense of touch by both physically and figuratively 'touching'. For example, we can physically touch leaves, tree bark, stones, the vegetables we prepare for dinner, clean clothes in the washing basket. Figuratively touching is more about sensing our own mood. How do I feel today? This also involves trust and the sense of life (see Chapter 7).

We use our sense of touch figuratively when meeting another person: our mood, choice of words and gestures are all woven into the conversation and experience. If our sense of touch is well developed, we can easily set boundaries between ourselves and the world. Someone with a healthy sense of touch is not afraid to be emotionally 'touched'; experiencing feelings and being emotionally 'moved' allows us to know our deepest self. The sense of touch helps us to understand, acknowledge and respect ourselves and others.

Touching is something we feel in different ways. Something can touch the skin, but our eyes can also touch or probe. We all know the saying: 'He undressed me with his eyes.' Anyone who has ever experienced this will agree how unpleasant this feels. Parents examine their children daily with their eyes, but what expression do we use? Is it positive or negative? Do our expressions show respect and honesty?

All children's experiences need to be processed and contemplated. Rest, time, attention and trust are all required to give children the right environment in which to process these experiences. Even though children may look as if they're doing nothing or are 'bored' when resting, they are probably hard at work. We should ensure daily routines include plenty of rest between activity, giving children the space to come from nothing to something.

Encouraging feelings of security and the sense of touch

The table below shows the qualities children require and those caregivers should foster in order to help children develop a strong sense of security.

Children require	Caregivers provide
Budding sense of self	Appropriate boundaries
Trust	Protection
Body perception	Availability/presence
Feeling	Consistency
Security	Leadership
Relaxation	Empathy
The right to exist	Nurture
Contentment	Giving children rest and space
Space to be absorbed by something	Attention
Feeling at home	Making room in our lives for children
Senses	Control

7. Two: Building Trust

All art forms are in the service of the greatest of all arts: the art of living.

Bertolt Brecht

Child	Parent/carer
Trust	Giving
1. 0–1 year old	
2. Sense of life (well-being and harmony)	
3. Surrender, daring to open up to someone or something	4. Being caring and sympathetic; watching, following, and mirroring children; talking and babbling with them, naming things
5. Distrust	6. Taking

Another building block that develops in the first year of life is trust. In the early months both parents and children are learning to adapt to each other. Are parents meeting the needs of their children, responding to signals such as the need for comfort, attention, care, dependability and predictability?

Verbal and non-verbal contact – through the skin, voice and shared experiences such as walks, meals and getting dressed – strengthen the attachment between parents and children, and children's ability to have faith in their caregivers. At changing time, caregivers can let babies know that they will be cleaned, massaged with cream or oil, and given a new nappy. Throughout the process, eye contact, tone of voice, volume and tempo are all centred on the infant. Although the baby may not understand exactly what's happening, the words and actions give peace and connection, building a bridge of faith between parent and child.

The sense of life

When we speak about the senses, we usually mean the five accepted senses of sight, touch, hearing, smell and taste. But, as outlined in Chapter 1, Rudolf Steiner described further senses, which allow us to look in more detail at the quality of experiences and the feelings of well-being, harmony and vitality. Am I in harmony with my surroundings? How do I feel, and where do I feel this? Exploring the sense of life will allow us to answer these questions. Every day, we sense whether we have slept well, how we connect with other people, and how we feel physically: Am I rested? Did I react with understanding or was I agitated? Am I hungry or thirsty? The sense of life, working closely with our other senses, lets us experience these feelings. In the first year of life, the foundations are laid for developing this sense, which requires care and attention throughout life, if we are to feel comfortable within ourselves – physically well, emotionally balanced and in harmony with the world around us.

The sense of life in the first year

Babies are completely dependent on their caregivers to keep them safe and provide for all their needs. They rely on us to react to signals they give about their state of comfort and happiness, which in turn allows them to have faith in themselves and in the world around them. In general, it's not long before new parents learn to recognise different types of crying and what they mean: one is asking for comfort, one for hunger, one for a dirty nappy, one for pain, and so on. Parents develop extremely sensitive relationships with babies, and can often instinctively judge what they require to be as comfortable as possible during their first year.

Parents must help babies become accustomed to the rhythm of waking and sleeping, night and day: rhythm and routine are golden rules. They must regulate the balance between warm and cool by providing and removing clothing appropriately. When babies feel uncomfortable, it's important that they sense their parents are doing everything possible to make them feel comfortable again. In this way, babies learn to surrender themselves to their body and their surroundings – to trust themselves and others.

Babies also need parents who can respond to their complete needs and be there in body and soul. For example, a one-year-old is out for a stroll with her father and sees a dog, but can't say the word 'dog' yet. She looks at her father as if to say, 'Don't we know that dog?' and is exceedingly happy when the father confirms with eye contact that she's right and says, 'Yes, that's our neighbours' dog. Hi Buster!' In this way the father inhabits the child's world and experiences it with her.

Often we experience the sense of life when our everyday routine is disrupted. This can be as simple as having lunch later than usual. When young children feel tired, hungry or out of sorts, their sense of life is disrupted. For example, a family with two young children aged one and three years old are on their way home from an outing with friends. Their train is late and both children are whining and crying; they should have been in bed an hour ago. Situations like this are stressful for parents, but if they understand why the children are reacting in this way and how significant this kind of disruption of routine is for young children, they can respond effectively. Instead of getting anxious or shouting, simply explaining that: 'It's late and the day is going a little differently today' and by singing, telling a story and staying calm, they will stay connected to their children. The children will surrender to their own inabilities because they know their parents will look after them. The parents will comfort and emotionally carry their children during this temporary disruption of their sense of life.

Separation anxiety

Between the ages of five months and three years, children go through different phases of seeking intimacy and distancing themselves during the process of individuation. Many babies between five and eight months develop what is termed 'separation anxiety'. In this important developmental phase, children first realise that something has gone, and they are anxious that it won't come back. Initially this 'something' is a parent, but it can also be a toy. Of course, the parent reappears after going to the kitchen, upstairs, or to collect their child from care after a day's work. By reappearing, an image grows in the child's mind, an image of the comforting parent, who lets the child know that they will always come back. Through reappearing reliably, and through peek-a-boo games, children develop the ability to conjure up the image of their parents when they are away. The same is true for objects.

Researchers believe that this recollection of images is the first known 'thought activity' of babies. Parents who can support their children in this developmental step contribute to the first building blocks in the process of individuation and the development of thought. In this stage of development it is important that parents are there for children, are available, predictable, sympathetic and can empathise with them. When children trust their parents and know that they will always return to offer comfort, the sense of life is restored, children stay bonded with themselves and their surroundings, and the process of healthy attachment evolves.

Fulfilling desires and setting boundaries

During the first years of life, babies are completely dependant on their parents, but as children grow up, their needs become more specific. For example, a toddler must learn that we sometimes go out for an ice cream in summertime, but that this is less likely during the rest of the year. In spring, as soon as the sun shines many kindergartners ask if they can go outside without their coats. Adolescents want to go out all three evenings over the weekend even when they have an exam on Monday. Children of all ages need parents to help them determine if these desires will contribute to a balanced and vitalising sense of life.

During my work as a kindergarten teacher, I met parents who felt that their child's needs were central to everything: if the child screamed, he should be allowed to scream; if he was hungry, he should be allowed to eat, completely disregarding the rhythm of the class. Fulfilling children's needs does not mean that we should raise princes and princesses and pander to their every desire. Children want to be part of their village. They want to get to know the 'rules' of that village so that they too can live in harmony, trust and understanding. They want to be part of 'us'. Children who are raised with healthy attachment may well grow up to be adults who behave like kings and queens, reigning with love and wisdom, and living happily ever after.

Play

Play is essential in caring for the sense of life. When children (and adults) play, harmony is restored, for example cradling, rocking, playing with hands and feet, peek-a-boo games, sitting on a rocking horse, circle games, fantasy games, crafting, drawing, playing football with friends, making music and so on. All activities that are predictable, and provide rhythm, repetition and order help to rebalance our sense of life.

Warmth

Every relationship needs warmth. People with a well-developed sense of touch, life, movement and balance will know which type of warmth is needed for which relationship (you hug your loved ones, you shake a doctor's hand).

In the process of healthy attachment both children and their caregivers need warmth to grow. A child who is unhappy because he is angry, has lost his favourite marble or is not allowed to play with the others, 'defrosts' when a parent is nearby offering warmth – not through symbiotically joining the child in his sorrow, but through attention, sympathy, trust and love at a fitting distance.

How parents can help

The attachment pyramid indicates that the sense of life relates to feelings of happiness and harmony, among others. The sense of life is an important companion for parents. When my own children were young, I physically experienced that after a broken night's sleep due to illness or teething, I felt less energy, patience and understanding towards them than when I was rested. When rested, parents have more confidence in life, feel more balanced within themselves and with the world around them, and can therefore provide healthier surroundings. Every parent has experienced the powerful interaction between themselves and their children; whether consciously or unconsciously, children copy the mood of their parents.

It can be useful for parents to look at their own sense of life: What gives me energy? In what surroundings do I feel comfortable? How much sleep and nourishment do I need? How do I stay healthy and balanced in a world with so many other pressures? Revisiting our own biographies and how our parents dealt with well-being, harmony, availability, comfort, body language and touch can be of interest and may bring unconscious patterns to the surface. These patterns can then be broken or changed through self-development or by seeking outside help, if required. The more parents can reflect on their own childhood and how their sense of life developed, the more they will be able to offer their own children.

Parents act as a bridge between young children and

the world. One way to reinforce this bridge is to 'mirror' actions and experiences with words, as in the nappy changing instance earlier (see p.55) and the example of seeing Buster the dog while on a walk. As babies grow older their world also grows, as does the 'mirror' parents use to reflect this world to their children. While walking in the park, a mother may talk to her son about the ducks in the water, a swan building a nest, a dog that barks. An eight-year-old girl may lose precious cards while playing a game at school; her parents may 'mirror' that certain games have rules, sometimes you lose and sometimes you win. A twelve-year-old boy may need a 'mirror' to help him navigate the digital world safely. Sometimes this requires strict boundaries.

Encouraging trust and the sense of life

The table below shows the qualities children require and those caregivers should foster in order to help children develop trust.

Children require	Caregivers provide
Confidence	Closeness
Physical contact	Pleasant skin contact
Eye contact	Positive facial expressions
Openness	Fulfilment of needs
Dependence	Reliability
Ability to surrender	Accommodating
Adaptability	Positive body language
Acceptance	Empathy
Receptibility	Care
Participation	Response
Daring to confide	Comfort

8. Three: Building Self-Confidence

Your authority is the ship on which your children ride, buoying them along as they test out possibilities and variations. It is what carries them until they master their own stroke...

Lea Page, *Parenting in the Here and Now*

Child	Parent/carer
Self-confidence	Support and compassion
1. 1–3 years old	
2. Sense of movement	
3. Exploring the world, dealing with separation anxiety, sharing joy and sadness, controlling emotions	4. Providing support and stimulation, compassion and understanding; letting children explore, naming things
5. (Insecurity)	6. (Indifference or over supervision)

The sense of (personal) movement

The sense of movement is one of the further senses we discussed earlier (see p.12). It encompasses physical movement as well as being 'moved' emotionally, moving with the thoughts of others and being able follow our own thoughts.

The sense of movement primarily develops in the first three years of life through learning to sit, crawl, walk, climb, fall and stand up again. During this time, young children are intent on exploring their world. The more confident they are, the more freedom they have to discover the world. Children come to understand the possibilities of movement within the boundaries set by their caregivers, and they learn by trial and error. Being allowed to fall allows children to experience, accept, and build up resistance in order to subsequently rise up again. To develop their sense of movement, children need plenty of 'Vitamin F' – F for frustration. A healthy amount of Vitamin F allows children to develop willpower and perseverance, which we see strongly when they learn to walk, reach a stubborn phase or learn to tie their own shoelaces. Learning to walk, in itself, is a gift for developing willpower. All children approach it in their own unique way, but it is never easy and requires great perseverance. Putting babies in 'walker' chairs does not aid in this process; it deprives them of learning in their own unique way and by trial and error.

The broader the opportunities and diversity of movement children are allowed to experience, the better developed their sense of movement will become, in all its characteristics – enabling them to grow into adults who have confidence in both their own inner movements (thoughts and emotions) and outer physical movements. Movement gives children freedom, not in an egocentric way, but through developing their self-confidence and attachment with their community; they become able to literally walk the paths of the village in which they live.

Through play and games, children experience the

gift of moving and 'being moved' together – ultimately we are all searching for attachment and a feeling of togetherness. Three-year-olds enjoy moving side by side, each absorbed in their own play. Adolescents enjoy playing games and sports together – I believe they look for a means of moving and 'being moved' collectively. The older the children, the more refined the movements and adjustments are to themselves and their surroundings. Everyone wants to find their own unique path in life. Allowing children freedom (and safety) of movement in their early years enables them to become open and free adults who are confident to walk their own path.

Exploring the world aged 1–3

During their first three years, toddlers start exploring and discovering the world through movement. They are curious by nature; everything is new. While they take the initiative to explore, they also look for the safe arms and security provided by their parents. If they are allowed to experience their personal need for movement within safe boundaries, their self-confidence grows. Typical to this phase is repetition: toddlers may open and close a kitchen cabinet repeatedly, and going up and down stairs is wonderful. Therefore it's hugely important that we're not always in a hurry!

This is the time of the 'terrible twos': children can seem quite stubborn, wanting to eat and get dressed by themselves – they want to be grown up! But they inevitably experience a struggle between wanting to do it by themselves and not being able to. The job of parents is tricky during this stage and power struggles lurk around many corners. Parents need to respond sensitively and try to maintain a healthy balance between leading and supporting.

Until they are around two-and-a-half to three, children experience their world as 'we': the bond with their parents is symbiotic and all encompassing. As they approach three, and these days at an increasingly young age (see Chapter 2, p.21), children first refer to themselves as 'I', a unique moment in the process of healthy attachment. During this phase, parents must be strong and clear, showing their children that they are the captains of the family ship. The roles must be clear: the parent is in charge, not the screaming child who's having a tantrum on the floor (see more on avoiding tantrums p.88).

Room to move

Being able to move about freely is a gift for children: walking in sand and on moss-covered stones or grass-covered paths, whether straight or curvy. Climbing, scrambling, walking and resting before moving off again. Free movement is priceless, whether within the boundaries of a playpen, lying on a rug, or walking around the house. Today, many babies spend hours at a time sitting in bouncy chairs, pushchairs or car seats, originally designed for safe travel. These have all become useful places to rest and sleep, but they are also confining. Movements such as pivoting around are not possible, and the process of learning to sit is accelerated. Being able to roll from back to front is an important experience as it lets babies discover all the directions in which their bodies can move. Of course, it is preferable that they experience this in their own time and not forced through outside stimuli. The only thing that truly stimulates children is imitating the people around them. If no one in a child's surroundings walks, the child will never learn to walk; babies copy other people in order to be part of the village.

Young children are highly sensitive to what happens in their surroundings. For example, in a preschool group, if one child cries a few others may follow: they 'move' with the crying child, to imitate and resonate with their companions. These young children are still developing their own inner, emotional life; they are still at one with the feelings of the group . Singing a song or gently rocking these children will restore their inner balance.

When children become rowdy and hyperactive, as young children often do (for example, if a storm is coming), it helps to give them an opportunity to move: go for a walk, do clapping games, jump up and down, all depending on their age and possibilities. Sometimes it helps to start whispering or talking very quietly. The golden rule is if the caregiver displays inner and outer peace, children will imitate and move with their leader.

Self-confidence through 'me doing'

Allowing room for 'me doing' is important for the sense of movement as it develops self-confidence. Children learn that they get better at things, such as getting dressed and eating, through practice. But of course, as we've already discussed, haste and young children do not work well together; time, rest, attention and predictability do. It can be useful to establish a routine that includes some relaxed times of day for 'me doing' and other times when parents help with getting dressed and eating, for example. If this is repeated regularly, children will accept and appreciate the boundaries.

How parents can help

Parents can give their children no greater gift than offering them room to explore freely and develop their sense of movement within safe boundaries. Activities such as taking a stroll, cycling, hanging the washing out to dry and singing together all boost children's self-confidence, as they realise they can do more and more by themselves. Through moving together, children's attachment to others and their self-confidence grows. Toddlers who go to playgroup, kindergarten or to play with a neighbour, thrive most if the parent can really let go and entrust their child to another carer.

During this phase, parents need to find a balance between being available and letting go. This is especially true for parents of 'terrible two-year-olds': how do I stay strong in the face of tantrums and stubbornness? It's helpful to remember that the child has just discovered a wonderful treasure: 'I am a unique human being! There is only one of me!'

Earlier I mentioned the image of the parent as captain of the ship. For children in this phase of childhood there is no gift as precious as a parent who takes on the role of captain and determines the ship's route, ensuring that the relationship between parent and child stays on an even keel and strengthening the bond between them.

The following example illustrates how deep the bond between a parent and a child can be, and reveal its influence through the sense of movement. A childcare practitioner spent the day watching a fourteen-month-old child crawling, climbing and clambering on play equipment in the garden. Each time he fell, he confidently got up and tried again; it was obvious that he enjoyed picking up the movement where he had left off. At the end of the day when his mother came to collect him, the little boy crawled confidently to the garden, climbed up a little ladder and slid down a slide without falling once. Due to the deep inner bond between parents and young children of this age and the confidence it gives children, they can sometimes do more when the parent is around than when alone.

The next example shows how children between three and five years old can be guided through their sense of movement. A father went to the supermarket with his two children aged three and five, who were running around the shop. The mission for their adventure was to choose dinner together. When they went to pick vegetables one child wanted broccoli while the other wanted carrots, and the father thought salad with tomatoes would be nice. So they loaded all these vegetables and more into their trolley. After that, choosing pudding was impossible! In the end, an irritated father and his crying children pushed an overflowing cart to the till. In the same supermarket another father with children of the same age told them that Mummy would be late home from work today so they were going to prepare dinner together to surprise her. The five year old jumped up and down in excitement! The father reminded them that Mummy loves spaghetti with tomato sauce and salad, so they went to find all the ingredients they needed to make Mummy's favourite dish. The eldest was allowed to put the tomatoes in a bag, the father weighed them, and the youngest chose the onions. They finished quickly and happily and before they knew it, they were on their way home.

The above examples illustrate that young children find it difficult to make decisions when given a lot of choice and no boundaries; when asked to act as individuals, their unguided senses of movement got mixed up. The second father linked cooking for Mummy to a feeling of 'we'; the children's sense of movement was guided by a more experienced parent so they could work together effectively.

I'm sure every parent is familiar with situations in which children are given too much freedom, which conversely results in a complete lack of it! Parents must find a healthy balance between guiding and supporting, between both watching children practise doing things by themselves and doing things for their child.

Adults and the sense of movement

Adults can develop their sense of movement by literally moving: in the garden, going for walks, playing sports, cycling, playing a musical instrument, etc. The same is true for adults as it is for children: the more freely we move, the more confident we become in ourselves and in the world around us.

We can also study our movements by considering: How do I walk? How do I put groceries in the trolley? How do I shake someone's hand? Through paying attention to these routine movements, we can do them consciously and make adjustments.

It may also be interesting to study the figurative side of the sense of movement: being moved or moving with other people. One of the best ways to practise this is in conversations with others: Can I interpret what is being said between the lines? Can I follow someone else's thought process? Can I feel where a conversation is going? Can I sense when a conversation should end? How freely do I deal with adversity in my life?

Encouraging self-confidence and the sense of movement

The table below shows the qualities children require and those caregivers should foster in order to help children develop self-confidence.

Children require	Caregivers provide
Self-confidence	Stimulation
Allowed to be self-centred	Space
Ability to ask for attention	Attention
Able to share feelings	Reaction
Allowed to be stubborn	Understanding
Discovering first 'I' experience	Letting go
Emotional dependence	Reliability
Exploring	Active listening
Giving and taking	Openness
Curiosity	Support
	Physical presence

9. Four: Building Independence

Only those without imagination flee in reality.

Loesje International

Child	Parent/carer
Independence	Strong and clear
1. 3–4 years old	
2. Sense of balance	
3. Aware that they can do things by themselves, saying 'I', being able to form an inner image of another person, concentration, giving and taking	4. Giving children more personal space, using the word 'I', setting boundaries without rejecting, giving clear guidance
5. Loneliness	6. Being vague

Sense of balance

The sense of balance is another of the further senses we have discussed (see p.12). It encompasses physical balance as well as inner emotional balance. If the building blocks of attachment are well developed and children have sufficient physical and inner stability, they will be able to stand independently on their own two feet. Depending on their age, they will be able to move independently through the world, both literally and figuratively.

As young children grow, language becomes increasingly important as the bridge between their inner and outer worlds. In their second year, in general, children start naming the world: pointing at things around them, which their caregivers then name. Earlier we mentioned the moment a child sees a dog and the parent recognises it and gives it a name (see p.57). The child registers that the word 'dog' means the neighbour's dog, then slowly starts to realise that the word 'dog' can also mean other dogs. Through language, children begin to develop a personal connection to the world, which they can increasingly discover. However, their sense of 'self' is still highly dependent on the feelings of others. Parents need to be clear and resolute during this phase, while also allowing room for movement and discovery.

Movement gives young children the experience of physical balance: walking through sand, mud, water, over forest paths and gravel; climbing and clambering, falling and getting up again. Children should be allowed to experience small discomforts, knowing that their caregiver is always there to comfort them when needed. Through developing their sense of balance, children are able to become more independent.

Repetition and play

As mentioned earlier (see p.46), young children love repetition. It allows them to experience predictability, which in turn builds inner balance. We can introduce repetition in any number of ways: looking at the same picture book over and over again, listening to stories or fairy tales that have repetition, playing the same game until children have processed or internalised its theme. Children's ability to concentrate also increases through play.

More and more of the adult world is imitated through children's own independent play: stacking bricks like a bricklayer, listening to a teddy bear's stomach like a doctor, building a garage for toy cars like the garage at home.

Memory

Children aged two-and-a-half to three years can remember past events or what happened earlier in the day, week or even longer. Memory is connected to sense experiences at this age – children make connections through smell or sounds. Asking toddlers what they did today makes no sense to them. It is only when they experience a feeling that they can connect with the past that they can remember. For example, before eating snack at preschool, the teacher sings a certain song; when having lunch at home with Mum, the child suddenly breaks into the song from preschool and says what happened during morning snack that day. In contrast, children aged 6–7 years are able to consciously remember something that has no presence in the current moment, but can be connected to an earlier experience.

The freer children are to develop this process of internalising images and experiences, being allowed to do this in their own time, the stronger the development of their inner sense of balance. Some prerequisites for this building block are: the environment in which children are raised is rich in experiential possibilities, which invite them to develop on various levels (language, maths, play, socially, emotionally, movement, nature, etc.); there are adults to learn from and peers to learn with; the environment is safe; there is rhythm, routine, order, structure; there are times to celebrate; experiences in the natural world; the home and outside worlds in which children live mirror and respect one another.

How parents can help

As parents we must give our children room to celebrate their independence within safe boundaries. Toddlers are just embarking on discovering themselves as individuals and we should respect this, patiently allowing them to take their time to develop their newly found independence. Folding the laundry takes ten times longer with a toddler than without, but notice what pleasure children experience in 'helping'!

As young children start to develop their own play and fantasy world, they learn to play by themselves, giving parents a little more time to do something for themselves (even if only for a few minutes at a time!). Sometimes it's helpful to tell children that you're busy doing a job and they can play nearby: developing a rhythm and habit of being together but acting independently – a continuation of habits formed from birth.

In my kindergarten I played the following game with a child who found it difficult to experience the boundary between himself and someone else. He found the difference between what was his and what was another child's difficult, and often called himself by his name instead of saying 'I'. In fact, he didn't come to develop his sense of self and understanding of 'I' until he was four-and-a-half years old. To help this child, I said and acted out the following verse with the group for several weeks. All the children enjoyed saying the verse and doing the actions, not just the boy with the particular need.

Round and round and round again.
This is straight, and this is bent.
This is a house, and this is an egg.
This is a ship, and this is a bridge.
The ship sails there, and comes back here.
I am here, and you are there.

Encouraging independence and the sense of balance

The table below shows the qualities children require and those caregivers should foster in order to help children to become independent.

Children require	Caregivers provide
Independence	Free space
Understanding	Letting go
Language	Patience
Self-consciousness	Trust
Freedom	Clarity
Sense of self – 'I'	Using the word 'I' in context
Imagination	Independence
Concentration	Boundaries

10. Five: Building Creativity

During play, children use their imaginations to create a world from within themselves. If they have many opportunities to play, they are flexing their cognitive muscles (so to speak), and will become creative thinkers for life.

Lou Harvey-Zahra, *Happy Child, Happy Home*

Child	Parent/carer
Creativity	Having confidence
1. 4–5 years old 2. All senses 3. Solving problems independently and with others, showing empathy, role play 5. Incapable	4. Having confidence in our children, letting go in full faith 6. Being fearful/anxious

The last building block – creativity – sits on top of the pyramid like a crown. From four years onwards children can be completely absorbed in their own unique play; not one child in this world plays the same game. Children who feel safely attached to their parents unconsciously experience the inner freedom of movement (sense of movement) and inner balance (sense of balance) to explore (sense of touch) their game in harmony (sense of life).

The interchange between children and their environment (friends, adults) continuously increases now that they can express themselves through language. Children start to understand more and more situations and imitate them in play. While toddlers play alongside their peers, slowly the desire and ability to play with other children grows. Children now have enough language to be able to play together for a longer length of time. They have developed a strong enough sense of self to take initiative, stand up for themselves and become more independent.

They want to solve their own problems: How do I fasten a mast to my boat? How can the couch become a train? How do I build an Eiffel Tower with my blocks? By solving problems through play, such as 'How do I build a den for me and my friends with these sheets and crates?' children develop new pathways of thinking. Later in life, these pathways will help with learning maths, tying shoelaces, making a bed: 'First I'll do this, then I'll do that and then that happens.'

Language becomes the instrument through which children can express their individual thoughts. The imagination is at its peak during these years. The world of fantasy is endless whether in the sandbox, on a balcony or in the play corner at home. Through play the sandbox is a desert, the balcony is a land far, far away and the play corner is a wonderful castle. Anything is possible, but children know that it's all 'make-believe'.

How parents can help

Giving children the confidence to become creative, and

allowing them to do this in their own way, is the greatest gift a parent can give. Creativity is most expressed through free play, whether imaginative role play, outdoor play, or play with construction materials or crafts. All forms of play can be creative, but for free play it is essential that children determine how to create their own games and do not have to follow directions given by adults. Children should be given the freedom to explore the world, to digest life's experiences and to discover and create their own unique imagination. Parents are welcome to come for a visit when invited into the child's castle, but playing together is not advisable as it disturbs the children's own free creative process. Parents must have faith in their children's ability to make their own play. Children who are healthily attached and are able to develop all the building blocks of the attachment pyramid will play their own games.

Encouraging independence and the sense of balance

The table below shows the qualities children require and those caregivers should foster in order to help children to become independent.

Children require	Caregivers provide
Imagination Initiative Role play All types of free play	Trust and confidence

Part 3.
Further Advice for Everyday Parenting

11. The Inner Working Model: Weaving the Bond

A child coming to earth can be compared to the launching of a ship. The journey through life offers a wealth of experiences but none are without danger: the ship may run aground in shallow water, stall in extreme heat, get caught in a storm, lose its way and be shipwrecked. The captain must battle with the elements of earth, air, fire and water to find safe passage.

Paul Biegel

Children are born into, grow up in and bond with the world around them. They gain many experiences, some wonderful but others not so positive. Through these experiences, they create an inner working model, often referred to as the reaction pattern that children build within themselves over the years: their reaction to the feelings and events they experience during childhood. When I first heard the words 'inner working model', I found them cold and abstract. I prefer to call them 'inner weaving'.

Inner weavings are made up of threads of experience, feelings, habits and thoughts. The resulting patterns are made from children's reactions to situations. Our lives are based on these inner weavings – they give us a foothold – but they are completely subconscious. They support us, but if patterns formed in childhood negatively influence how we live our adult lives, they can get in the way.

For example, a toddler discovered that there are lots of yummy things in the supermarket that she likes to eat. She watched time and time again how her parents took things from the shelves and put them in the shopping trolley. She was only young and lived through imitation, so she thought, 'I want to do this too, I want to put all those yummy things in the trolley!' But Mum and Dad didn't like it when she put things she liked in. To her, this was incomprehensible. She began to cry, started a tantrum and then, all of a sudden, she was allowed to put what she wanted in the cart. Mum and Dad's voices sounded different from usual, though, and their faces were red, but she didn't understand: she was allowed to put something yummy in the cart, but her parents were still angry. And then they also said, 'OK, just this once! Next time you have to listen to me!' The reaction to the situation and the feeling this aroused in the child formed an inner weaving pattern made up of two parts:

1. The expectation in relation to the other party (parents): if I cry and throw a tantrum, my parents will let me put those yummy biscuits in the trolley.
2. The expectation in relation to herself: if I get angry, I get what I want and I get control over the world that I want so much to understand.

For young children, having control over the world is connected with understanding it. They don't understand why their parents can put something in the trolley but they can't. They don't understand the situation and can't get control over it, but control returns if they get angry and throw a tantrum. So throwing a tantrum does the trick! In this way children develop an inner weaving pattern which tells them that throwing tantrums and whining work as a way of gaining control.

Breaking internal patterns

Our inner weaving patterns change with new experiences. If the supermarket scene had transpired in the following way, it would have had a positive effect on the young child's inner weaving:

A father took his three-year-old son shopping. The man knows that supermarkets are full of temptations for youngsters and that his son thinks, 'When Daddy puts something in the trolley, I want to imitate him!' The man picked a trolley with a child seat and put his son in. He was now captain of the ship (trolley) and in control of where the ship and its cargo (the child) were going. He gave unbreakable items such as paper towels and tissues to his son to put in the trolley. He led by example and his son copied, allowing the boy to act according to his age and level of understanding.

Children (and parents) will react to situations such as the scene above according to what they have experienced in the past and the inner weavings created thereby. If safe inner patterns have been established, children will interpret new social situations as being secure. If children experience situations in which they don't feel safe, their inner weavings will develop accordingly and they will interpret new situations as being unsafe. It is in these stressful moments that we can best observe and assess the attachment process.

Let's now think about how this applies to parents. Everyone feels stressed sometimes, especially when we don't get enough sleep due to young children teething, having bad dreams, etc. Fatigue disrupts the sense of life. Some people become irritable, others become quiet and closed off, others become emotional and raise their voices or lose their patience. For example, an exhausted mum might feel emotional and raise her voice, saying, 'I've tried so hard to make today fun. I read to you when I really wanted to go to sleep. I cooked a special meal and you didn't eat it. I never do anything right!' Within this mother's inner weaving pattern there may be thread that came from always wanting to do everything perfectly, which will have caused her to always push herself to the limit in childhood. This thread appears again with fatigue or stress. Through self-awareness and self-education, parents can work on and change these threads.

12. Educating the Will

Childlike imagination paves the way for creativity later in social life and in a career.

Bernard Lievegoed

All children have a natural urge and desire to become adults. Young children have so much to learn – walking, talking, thinking – preferably all within the first three years of life. Never again in our lives are so many milestones reached in such a short space of time. Children need willpower to achieve these goals and it's important that they have ambitions in life. Before this can be manifested, parents and children must travel a long and significant road together, and there are many 'helpers' along the way who can assist in raising our little bundles of will.

When I taught in a kindergarten, some parents, arriving at school for the first time, would tell me their children were very 'strong willed', which usually meant the parents felt powerless to steer their children's desires; they found their children's will to be stronger than their own. For example, after enrolling his four-year-old daughter at kindergarten, a father collected her coat, hat and shoes and started getting ready to leave. The father asked the young girl to put her coat on, but she didn't want to wear it and threw it on the floor. The father picked it up and asked her once again to put on the coat. The same situation continued and before long the father was angry, the child was screaming and the coat was still on the floor. Because he had *asked* his child to put on her coat, she thought the action was negotiable. If he had simply put on his own coat, leading by example, the child would have imitated him: 'Let's *both* put on our coats.'

If a mother says to a three-month-old baby, 'I want you to sleep through the night from now on because I'm tired,' she doesn't expect it to actually happen and most likely nothing will. If she tells a toddler not to throw tantrums in the supermarket any more, most likely nothing will happen either – but she might expect it to.

If she decides to work on sleep and eating routines, taking into account the knowledge that some children take longer to adjust to this process than others, she's already well on the way to guiding the child's will. If she understands that toddlers imitate everything we do, including putting groceries in the supermarket trolley, she is well on the way to understanding how to avoid tantrums.

Four helpers in educating the will

There are four loyal helpers that help parents and caregivers to raise children. They are: imitation, establishing routines, respect and imagination. These 'will helpers' are directly connected to healthy attachment. Children walk and talk because they *imitate* the adults around them. *Habits* and routine give children rest and regularity and therefore a feeling of safety – one of the building blocks for healthy attachment. Raising children with *respect* means we approach each child with deep wonder and admiration of their unique self and their potential in life. All parents, caregivers and teachers need *imagination* and humour in order to develop positive and loving connections with children.

1. Imitation

When children imitate, they copy exactly what their parents do with complete trust and devotion. Children imitate everything they observe parents doing – movement, way of walking, intonation, feeling, thinking – whether consciously or subconsciously. This sometimes moves us, and sometimes confronts us with ourselves. In their movements, intonation and habits children show what subconscious influence parents and caregivers have. Below are a few examples:

A preschool teacher had the habit of pulling up her tights around her knees each time she stood up. One day she realised that the children all made a similar movement when they got up. A terribly embarrassed mother told the story that her toddler often said the word 'shit', and only then did she notice that she often said the word without realising. A kindergarten teacher and a mother noticed that her son had recently started to limp and drag one leg. The mother took the child to the doctors and was told nothing was wrong. A few days later, the mother saw a man walking across the schoolyard, limping and slightly dragging his leg. After enquiring why, he told her that he was recovering from a broken leg. Apparently, watching the man had made such an impression on the boy that he subconsciously imitated his walk.

Prerequisites for imitation

First of all, children must be able to imitate. Those who are born deaf will never be able to imitate language and intonation. But children must also want to imitate. Those who are using all their energy to recover from a high fever will probably not be interested in imitating the actions of a song; they are temporarily 'closed for essential maintenance' – not open to their surroundings.

Imitation requires an example from parents or teachers, preferably one that encourages children to give themselves freely and with love. Trust in the world, in parents and caregivers and in themselves forms the foundation for imitation. Parents and caregivers must provide examples of movement, habits, language and mood with love and affection. Of course, this love and affection must be genuine, not forced or artificial. Making mistakes is part of life. Every parent makes mistakes and children don't ask for perfection, only for authenticity and purity. They ask their parents to show them how to become a human being: 'Show me how you handle happiness, sorrow and disappointment, so that I know how to respond to these feelings when I grow up.'

Imitation means being moved by something someone else does; being inspired by another person to follow their intonation, expression, posture, gesture or anything else that can be imitated. Children don't think about this process; it's completely unconscious. When children imitate, their inner world resonates with their outer world (parents, family, classmates), much like the strings of a musical instrument resonate when plucked. The sound of an instrument depends upon the person playing it and changes in different hands. Not one human body is the same as another and people are never 'tuned' in exactly the same way. Likewise, children resonate and imitate in their own unique manner. In the example of the kindergartner who limped, this particular imitation was unique to that child. If the whole class had begun walking this way it would have been extremely unusual!

Children can only imitate what they have experienced (consciously or subconsciously) and their ability to observe grows as their senses mature. Some children will imitate certain things while others will not; they subconsciously decide what to imitate. For me, this individuality makes each child a mystery; children have their own unique secrets and plans for the future.

2. Habits

Habits form from our own inner world and are created in the past. We don't have to think about them; they are just there. We walk because we know how, we drink a glass of water in our own way, we climb stairs so uniquely that our family members know who's coming. If we had to think before doing everything, we would never get anywhere. We do many things out of habit. Habits are like paths in a forest that we have followed many times. Even if we haven't walked them in years, we will find our way because, instinctively, we know where we're going. Habits are formed in our memory.

Habits also build a foundation of trust, and provide security and safety. Imitation is done unconsciously, but a parent may consciously try to instil certain habits in their children in order to teach them something. For example, coats belong on the coat rack, not on the floor. We look after our belongings and we want to live in an orderly home.

Habits are not easy to change. They become engraved in our memory and seem to stay there. A habit can be tackled by trying to avoid thinking about it or by creating another habit in its place. Habits evolve with a family.

A mother once told me that her children found out about sweet treats when they were toddlers. A kind neighbour had given them some and they wanted to have more. The mother decided to buy some 'good' treats at the local organic food store. Each day, the children asked for treats and, although 'healthier' than other alternatives, this mother did not want eating them to become a habit. She decided to do the following: every Wednesday and Saturday at 3 pm, it was 'treat time' when she gave the children a small bowl of raisins, an apple and a few chocolate buttons. These children, who are now grown up, look back on these happy memories with nostalgia, and no one can remember when these 'treat times' stopped. At some point the habit was lost in memory.

Children like habits such as these because they give them support and bring rhythm and structure to their lives. But even good habits should not become compulsive; it's healthy for children as well as adults to relax once in a while and let go of routine. Some children can handle this better than others, but it helps develop flexibility and tolerance. Holidays provide a good opportunity to relax our routines – with no work or school to attend we can get up later, enjoy a relaxed breakfast and rest more. Children aged nine to twelve love having a pyjama day – staying in their pyjamas all day long and doing whatever they like, not even eating at the table. After holidays and days like this, getting back into our normal, more structured routines can be refreshing.

However, not all children cope well with changes in rhythm. Parents will have to decide for themselves what's best for their children. The most important thing is that parents are there for them, and children feel sufficient predictability to feel safe. Children will only feel at ease in their surroundings, and will only be able to bond with themselves and others in a healthy way, if they feel completely safe.

3. Respect

When people come to visit a newborn baby, they often automatically lower their voice. A certain tenderness affects everyone in the room and even the toughest people seem to soften when they see or hold a newborn. They are showing their deep respect for this new life. Respect is one of the greatest wonders of humanity.

Young children carry respect as a precious possession deep within themselves. They want to demonstrate and recognise it, and it becomes evident in the way they interact with the world: the way a toddler who's just learning to walk places her feet on earth; the way my one-and-a-half-year-old son stroked his newborn sister and gave her a pinecone! Later in life we see this respect in the way loved ones caress each other, or in the way my grandmother swept breadcrumbs from the table, caught them in her hand and scattered them in the garden for the birds to enjoy. Respect makes us aware of the wider 'spiritual' world around us. It's a pleasure to watch people act out of respect; we sense that their actions are just; respect confirms, and goes hand-in-hand with awe and admiration.

Families live together with respect for one another and parents let children know that they are aware of that other world, the world that is larger than is visible at this moment; that other world in which the present, past and future join. Respect contributes to the foundations of moral development, helping us do what is right and become human beings. Respect cannot be learned, as a habit is learned, but must be demonstrated through living.

Respect can act as a link in the process of attachment. When children feel that their parents respect them as individuals, when they understand that they may freely encounter others, respect can act as a bridge between their inner and outer worlds, which they feel confident to cross.

4. Imagination

Imagination, or fantasy, brings creative power and new possibilities. When raising children, we can use fantasy to connect the physical and the imaginative, or unseen, worlds. Young toddlers don't yet have a rich imagination. They play through imitating their surroundings, thereby getting to know the world in which they live. In contrast, preschoolers and kindergartners have vivid imaginations, which they use in fantasy play. Their creative powers are endless: everything can become anything, before changing again. But their play does not dissolve the boundaries between the real and fantasy worlds – they know their play is imaginary. Imagination gives children freedom and is positive as long as it stays within healthy limits. It allows children to withdraw into their own world in which everything is possible, while still being connected to the here and now.

Fantasy and creativity are powered by an abundance of vitality. At the end of a long week, I can no longer write a good story. I have to recharge my battery before I can become creative again. It's important that children get enough sleep, so they wake up full of the energy that they will need during the day to live and be creative. In the attachment pyramid (see p.39) we saw that the sense of life is related to feelings of well-being and harmony, both of which stem from vitality. Children and adults who feel safely attached have enough vitality to be creative, giving them an extra level in life. This is particularly apparent in resilient, robust children.

Giving warning before ending free play

A child will know full well that a blue cloth may be water in play, but when playtime is over and the cloth is folded up, it is just a blue cloth again. The blue water belongs in the child's fantasy world, the blue cloth in the child's conscious world. The imagination that children experience in play should remain in the fantasy world and not become part of the children's consciousness. Children need time to let go of their fantasy worlds – to steer the boat they are sailing in on the blue water back to land. If they are asked to stop playing too abruptly, they will protest vehemently. Adults should warn them that they have 'five minutes' before it's time to tidy up. This helps children orientate themselves in time through predictability and trust.

Truth and lies: do young children lie?

Not one child has the same imagination. Imagination is a creative force that comes from within and shows involvement. A child's unique personality becomes visible through imagination. Almost anything is possible – the real world, the magical world, the fantasy world – they all intermingle.

Until about six or seven years of age, children are not conscious of a boundary between themselves, their parents, their friends and the world around them. They see their world as a totality, a whole that belongs together, with them at the centre. When I taught in kindergarten, the younger children often thought I lived at school and had a bedroom somewhere. They hadn't yet realised that I wasn't 'part of the school'. Many of them also thought I knew everything about their world: their pets, their grandparents etc. Because they experience their world as one, they feel that their imagination belongs to them. Fantasy is something children play with. Morality doesn't develop until after the sixth or seventh year, which is why young children cannot consciously lie, but they can 'play with fantasy' as the following example illustrates:

A little girl who had just turned four went to stay with her grandmother and took her doll, which could 'tell stories'. Every day at teatime, Grandmother gave the little girl a biscuit. These biscuits were so delicious, Grandmother suddenly found that the tin was almost empty. Although the little girl had crumbs on her cheeks, she still said, 'My doll ate the biscuits.'

In her fantasy world, maybe the doll ate the biscuit; young children cannot distinguish between truths and untruths. It is important that caregivers are genuine and honest if we wish to educate the imagination and create boundaries for overactive imaginations. We must live the truth and have built our own inner boundaries between reality and fantasy. If we are truthful, children can imitate and internalise our example. Reprimanding or punishing young children can be counterproductive. Children need recognition that their imagination is developing, and they need help to control this force to prevent it from taking over their imaginative playground.

Around the age of seven the imagination changes, as does children's play. Around the age of nine even more doors to the fantasy and magical world close and children discover that Father Christmas, the Easter Bunny and the Tooth Fairy all belong to a fantasy world.

13. Unhealthy Attachment

When you're scared but you still do it anyway,
that's brave.

Neil Gaiman, *Coraline*

No one can be one hundred per cent healthily attached. Somewhere in everyone's inner weaving, a thread will become knotted or unravelled, and this is completely normal. But when children suffer disruptions to the attachment process, more serious bonding disorders may arise, which we'll discuss in this chapter. During my time as a kindergarten teacher I met children who had been so damaged through the attachment process that they could no longer live at home nor stay with us in class, but had to be admitted to a psychiatric ward for children. Of course, every situation is unique.

A number of terms are used to label the various attachment problems. In the DSM-IV (Diagnostic and Statistical Manual of Mental Disorders – a classification system for mental disorders), experts described 'reactive attachment disorder' in infants and young children and distinguished between 'inhibited' and 'disinhibited' forms. In the DSM-V, these are now described as two different disorders: 'reactive attachment disorder' and 'disinhibited social engagement disorder'. Dutch Professor Riksen-Walraven distinguishes between the ambivalent type (inhibited) and fearful-ambivalent type (uninhibited). Experts also speak of 'disoriented attachment' in children. I have chosen the following terms for the three types of attachments disorders seen in children:

The *anxious-ambivalent* type: children with this disorder anxiously keep contact with their caregiver and do not explore. They are often noticeably dependent and panic instantly, saying they can't do something alone. They are afraid of new things and display cut-and-run and clamp behaviour if a trusted person (temporarily) leaves. The attachment figure is not always available to these children, who don't know where they stand with their parent or caregiver. Sometimes they are allowed on the caregiver's lap, and at others they may be pushed off in anger. Sometimes, in similar situations, they are given a hug and a compliment, while the next time they may be slapped and snapped at. Caregivers are inconsistent in their actions towards these children.

The *anxious-avoidance* type: these children explore their surroundings but barely keep contact with their attachment figure. They tend to actively look away, do not engage in eye contact and may walk off. Children with this disorder stay at arm's length, show little emotional expression and tend to be austere. They 'have to do everything alone', are seemingly independent and tend to fight. Their underlying fear is suppressed or dissociated. One of the most distinctive characteristics in the relationship between these caregivers and children is that caregivers have little or no physical contact with their children. Contact between them is business-like, and caregivers are quickly irritated and not in tune with the needs of their children.

The *disorganised attachment* type: these children alternate between flee and fight. If running away is no longer possible, they become numb. The attachment figure is unpredictable or disconnected in their relationship with their children, who experience role confusion between offender, victim and rescuer, both within themselves and with the perpetrator (caregiver). These children have often experienced traumatic situations such as (sexual) abuse or domestic violence in their close vicinity or towards themselves.

The attachment pyramid and insecure attachment

The attachment pyramid summarises the relationship between the senses, what caregivers can offer children and what children require to grow up in healthy attachment. The building blocks for the bodily senses form the foundation of our existence as symbolised by the pyramid. Children who experience insecure attachment lack sufficiently strong foundations; cracks form and their existence wobbles. Below, the senses are described in relation to children who have not been able to create healthy bonds. Parents and caregivers are asked to provide the foundation for each sense and attachment building block. Young children are completely dependent on the world and people around them; they are still working on building their existence and identity. Once again, the senses are linked to age.

Safety, fear and the sense of touch (0–1)

The continued absence of a feeling of basic safety and a lack of necessities such as food, warmth, clothing and shelter will result in disorders: children will not feel safe in their surroundings, will not be able to feel 'at home' within themselves and therefore will not be able to develop self-confidence. The reaction to this neglect is fear, which impedes healthy development. Children who do not feel safe desperately need our help.

Children show/are	Caregivers show/are
Apathy	Emotionally absent
Indifference	Seriously ill
Fear	Unpredictable
Dissatisfaction	Shortcomings
Tense	Unable to provide safety
Chaotic	Agitated
Unstructured	No structure
Anxious	Too much/too little stimulation
Agitated	Unsupportive
Hyperactive	Abuse
Weak	No physical contact
Lacking energy	Neglect

Trust, distrust and the sense of life (0-1)

Children whose sense of life has been neglected, whether for short or longer periods of time, distrust themselves and their surroundings. These children can feel so insecure, they don't dare submit to exploring their bodies and environment. They are afraid to loose themselves in play, games or exploration.

Children show/are	Caregivers show/are
Closed off	Changeable
Avoid contact	No interaction
Tendency to look away	Overwhelmed
No devotion	No influence
Distrust	Abandonment
Do not conform	Not in tune with their child
Rejection	Menacing
Clingy	Unpredictable
Superficial contact	Negative body language

Self-confidence, insecurity and the sense of movement (1-3)

Insecurely attached children are either too independent or too dependent. They either don't explore the world around them, or they run away. Those who are wise have learned that they are alone in life and must do everything themselves in order to survive. Their instinct for activity does not fit with their age or their stage of development. They can also cling to their caregivers, show aggressive resistant behaviour, bite, hit, demand continuous attention or show passive behaviour.

Children show/are	Caregivers show/are
Insecure	Distrust
Greedy	Rigid
Unsatisfied	Too little contact
Aggressive	Compulsive
Violent	Not available
Jealous	Rejection
Passive	Insulting
Independent	Dominant
Don't listen	Don't listen
Clingy	Changeable
Egocentric	Apathy
Purposeless	Too little attention

Independence, loneliness and the sense of balance (4–5)

Caregivers who are manipulative, hyperactive, provoking, forceful, and who limit space to develop personal identity, prevent their children from developing a sense of balance. These children have no direction and don't know who's the captain of their ship. They take either too little or too much room. These children can recede into powerlessness and show little emotion.

Children show/are	Caregivers show/are
Lonely	Not present
Stubborn	Authoritative
Rigid	Overbearing
Deceitful	Detached
Dependent	Impatient
Lack of concentration	No continuity
Fear of failure	Insulting
Insecure	Difficult to please
Ambivalent	Insecurity
Power struggles	Unable to let go
Manipulative	Don't set boundaries
Compulsive control	

Lack of creativity, powerlessness (4–5)

Cracks in the final building block arise when caregivers show no trust towards their children, who then feel completely powerless. This disorder is the result of neglect of all the underlying building blocks.

Children show/are	Caregivers show/are
Powerless Manipulative	Lack of trust

How caregivers can help

All these children need caregivers and/or social workers who are able to objectively bear and work with the attachment disorder. Children with attachment disorders needs caregivers who are extremely strong emotionally and will not be disconcerted by children who transmit mixed signals. For example, a child may want to sit on the caregiver's lap and be dependent one moment, but then yells, screams, hits and kicks the next. It is up to the caregiver to remain objective, meaning: don't be overjoyed when the child wants to sit on our lap and don't be angry when the child kicks and screams. Sometimes people can be so incredibly damaged that healing doesn't seem possible at that moment. However, I am a firm believer in the 'education of hope': I am convinced that every human being can believe that they are loved somewhere by someone, and that someone wants to show them what healthy attachment is.

I found inspiration in the following text when working with children with attachment disorders in my kindergarten class:

> Play and playing means entering the world of art, social art, and can only be practised with our most dear and vulnerable possession, our body.
>
> Triskel, Apeldoorn

14. The More Securely Attached the Better

A happy home is more than only a roof over your head, it's a foundation under your feet.

Amish proverb

Children who grow up with healthy attachment, and are able to develop according to the attachment pyramid, can become well bonded within themselves and with the world around them, growing into strong, confident adults.

I urge all caregivers to examine their own biographic inner weavings and to enjoy the colours and patterns that life has given them. But I also urge everyone to look for any frayed edges and knots in order to recognise work that still needs to be done. The verse on 'Childhood' from the International Joint Alliance Working Group (see p.14) will come true if we caregivers can take up this challenge of love for the world, each other and ourselves. We will then be able to build a world in which every soul can be healthily attached, genuine and authentic – a world that is good for our children and for every human being.

REFERENCES AND FURTHER READING

REFERENCES

Ainsworth, M.S., Belle, S.M., & Stayton, D.J. (1974) 'Infant-mother attachment and social development: Socialisation as a product of reciprocal responsiveness to signals' in M.P.M. Richards (Ed.) (1974) *The Integration of the Child into the Social World*, Cambridge University Press, London

Ainsworth, M.S., et al. (1978) *Patterns of Attachment: A Psychological Study of the Strange Situation*, Lawrence Erlbaum Associates, USA

Anderson, C. A., & Bushman, B. J. (2002) 'Human aggression', *Annual Review of Psychology*, vol.53, pp.27–51

Bakker, T. (2005) *Hechting in beeld*, www.123people.nl, via http://www.aitnl.org/hechtinghandout.pdf

—, (2008) *Zie je mij?*, www.123people.nl, via http://www.wereldkinderen.nl/site.php

Berkhout, L., Dolk, M. & Goorhuis-Brouwer, S. (2010) 'Teachers' views on psychosocial development in children from 4 to 6 years of age', *Educational & Child Psychology*, vol.27, no.4

Bijloo, M. (2002) *Hechting*, Medische Sectie Antroposofische Vereniging Nederland, Netherlands

—, (2004) in Niemeijer, M.H., Gastkemper, M., & Kamps, F.H.M. (Ed.) (2004) *Ontwikkelingsstoornissen bij kinderen: Medisch-psychologische begeleiding en behandeling* (Third revised edition), Koninklijke Van Gorcum, Netherlands

Bowlby, J. (1969) *Attachment and Loss, Vol.1: Attachment*, Penguin, London

—, (1975) *Attachment and Loss, Vol.2: Separation*, Penguin, London

—, (2005) *The Making and Breaking of Affectional Bonds (Routledge Classics)*, Routledge, London

Boszormenyi-Nagy, I. & Krasner, B. R. (1986) *Between Give and Take: A Clinical Guide to Contextual Therapy*, Brunner/Mazel, New York

Buber, M. (2002) *The Way of Man: According to the Teaching of Hasidim*, Routledge, London

Cyr, C., Euser, E.M., Bakermans-Kranenburg, M.J. & Van IJzendoorn, M.H. (2010) 'Attachment security and disorganization in maltreating and high-risk families: A series of meta-analyses', *Development and Psychopathology*, no.22, pp.87–108

IJzendoorn, M.H. van (1992) 'Intergenerational Transmission of Parenting: A Review of Studies in Non-Clinical Populations', *Developmental Review*, vol.12, pp.76–99

Kennedy, M.M. (2010) 'Attribution Error and the Quest for Teacher Quality', *Educational Researcher*, vol.39, no.8, pp.591–598

Riksen-Walraven, M. (1983) 'Mogelijke oorzaken en gevolgen van een (on)veilige eerste hechtingsrelatie. Een overzicht aan de hand van een model', *Kind en Adolescent*, vol.4, pp.23–44

—, (1983) 'Het belang van de eerste gehechtsheidsrelatie', *Kind en Adolescent*, vol.4, 23–44

—, (2000) *Tijd voor kwaliteit in de kinderopvang* (Inaugural speech, University of Amsterdam) Vossiuspers AUP, Amsterdam

—, (2004) 'Pedagogische kwaliteit in de kinderopvang. Doelstelingen en kwaliteitscriteria' in M.H. van IJzendoorn, L.W.C. Tavecchio & J.M.A. Riksen-Walraven (2004) *De kwaliteit van de Nederlandse kinderopvang*, Boom, Amsterdam

Riksen-Walraven, M. & Albers, E.M. (2008) *High quality child care and education for the youngest: A key role for the caregivers*, Paper presented at the Second International Conference on Early Childhood Education, March 6–7, 2008, Arnhem, Netherlands

Steiner, R. (1996) *The Education of the Child*, Anthroposophic Press, USA

—, (2003) *Soul Economy: Body, Soul and Spirit in Waldorf Education*, Steiner Books, USA

FURTHER READING

Anschütz, M. (1995) *Children and Their Temperaments*, Floris Books, Edinburgh

Burkhard, G. (1997) *Taking Charge: Your Life Patterns and Their Meaning*, Floris Books, Edinburgh

Harvey-Zahra, L. (2014) *Happy Child, Happy Home: Conscious Parenting and Creative Discipline*, Floris Books, Edinburgh

—, (2015) *Creative Discipline, Connected Family: Transforming Tears, Tantrums and Troubles While Staying Close to Your Children*, Floris Books, Edinburgh

Kiel-Hinrichsen, M. (2006) *Why Children Don't Listen: A Guide for Parents and Teachers*, Floris Books, Edinburgh

Gelitz, P. (2015) *The Seven Life Processes: Understanding and Supporting Them in Home, Kindergarten and School*, WECAN, USA

Kutik, C. (2010) *Stress-Free Parenting in 12 Steps*, Floris Books, Edinburgh

Köhler, H. (2013) *Working with Anxious, Nervous and Depressed Children*, Waldorf Publications, USA

Lievegoed, B. (2005) *Phases of Childhood: Growing in Body, Soul and Spirit*, Floris Books, Edinburgh

Neuschütz, K. (2013) *Children's Creative Play: How Simple Dolls and Toys Help Your Child Develop*, Floris Books, Edinburgh

Page, L. (2015) *Parenting in the Here and Now: Realizing the Strengths You Already Have*, Floris Books, Edinburgh

Schoorel, E. (2004) *First Seven Years: Physiology of Childhood*, Rudolf Steiner College Press, USA

—, (2016) *Managing Screen Time: Raising Balanced Children in the Digital Age*, Floris Books, Edinburgh

—, (2017) *Warmth: Nurturing Children's Health and Wellbeing*, Floris Books, Edinburgh

Soesman, A. (2006) *Our Twelve Senses: How Healthy Senses Refresh the Soul*, Hawthorn Press, UK

Solter, A. (1998) *Tears and Tantrums: What to do When Babies and Children Cry*, Shining Star Press, USA

—, (2013) *Attachment Play: How to Solve Children's Behavior Problems with Play, Laughter and Connection*, Shining Star Press, USA

—, (2001) *The Aware Baby*, Shining Star Press, USA

—, (1989) *Helping Young Children Flourish*, Shining Star Press, USA

Parenting in the Here and Now
Realizing the Strengths You Already Have

Lea Page

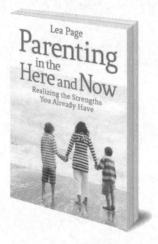

Being a good parent doesn't mean being perfect, learning complex theories or finding another twelve hours in the day. *Parenting in the Here and Now* offers a refreshingly different way. Rather than striving for – and failing to reach – a frustrating ideal, parents can start from where they are right now, and enjoy a more harmonious family life almost immediately.

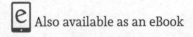 Also available as an eBook

florisbooks.co.uk

Managing Screen Time
Raising Balanced Children in the Digital Age

Edmond Schoorel

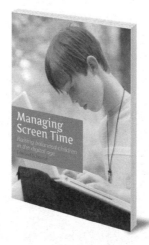

Screens and digital devices are everywhere in our modern world and it's becoming increasingly common for even very young children to regularly use tablets and smart phones.

This thought-provoking book offers a comprehensive overview of the pros and cons, to help parents make their own choices. It explores the health effects of screen time as well as the benefits of new technology, aiming to empower parents to find their own balance.

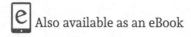 Also available as an eBook

florisbooks.co.uk

Happy Child, Happy Home
Conscious Parenting and Creative Discipline

Lou Harvey-Zahra

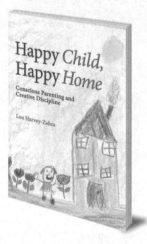

This practical and inspiring book introduces 'conscious parenting' as a new way of helping any family home become more harmonious. Lou Harvey-Zahra, an experienced parenting coach and teacher, draws her inspiration from a Steiner-Waldorf background, and offers candid advice for taking a clear look at family life, identifying what's not working, and exploring new ideas for improving relationships.

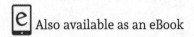 Also available as an eBook

florisbooks.co.uk

Creative Discipline, Connected Family

Transforming Tears, Tantrums and Troubles
While Staying Close to Your Children

Lou Harvey-Zahra

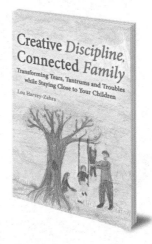

How can parents find effective ways of managing their children's behaviour, while maintaining closeness and trust in the family? With numerous examples and commonly asked questions, this is a helpful guide for parenting children from toddler to twelve years old from the author of the bestselling *Happy Child, Happy Home*.

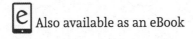 Also available as an eBook

florisbooks.co.uk

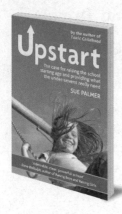 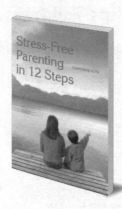 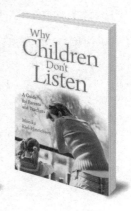
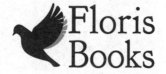